Cure Headaches Naturally

Top Tips to Keep Headaches under Control

By: Anne Higgins

9781681275086

PUBLISHERS NOTES

Disclaimer – Speedy Publishing LLC

This publication is intended to provide helpful and informative material. It is not intended to diagnose, treat, cure, or prevent any health problem or condition, nor is intended to replace the advice of a physician. No action should be taken solely on the contents of this book. Always consult your physician or qualified health-care professional on any matters regarding your health and before adopting any suggestions in this book or drawing inferences from it.

The author and publisher specifically disclaim all responsibility for any liability, loss or risk, personal or otherwise, which is incurred as a consequence, directly or indirectly, from the use or application of any contents of this book.

Any and all product names referenced within this book are the trademarks of their respective owners. None of these owners have sponsored, authorized, endorsed, or approved this book.

Always read all information provided by the manufacturers' product labels before using their products. The author and publisher are not responsible for claims made by manufacturers.

This book was originally printed before 2014. This is an adapted reprint by Speedy Publishing LLC with newly updated content designed to help readers with much more accurate and timely information and data.

Speedy Publishing LLC

40 E Main Street, Newark, Delaware, 19711

Contact Us: 1-888-248-4521

Website: http://www.speedypublishing.co

REPRINTED Paperback Edition: 9781681275086:

Manufactured in the United States of America

DEDICATION

This book is dedicated to my best buddy, Cynthia. Through every up and down, I promise to always be with you as you have always been with me.

TABLE OF CONTENTS

Chapter 1 - The Definition and Classifications of Headaches

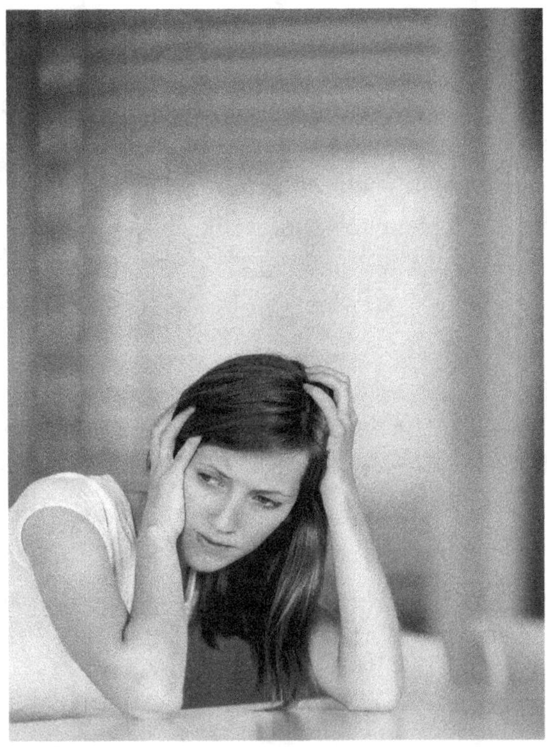

Everyone knows what a headache feels like. The pain can take many forms. For example, your head being trapped in vise; an angry blacksmith hammering on the inside of your skull; or maybe you just feel like your head is about to explode from the pressure building inside of it. You hold your head, search for a dark room, and wonder: why does my head hurt like this?

Although it often feels like your brain is swelling or your skull is pounding, the brain and the skull are actually incapable of feeling pain. So, what part of your head is it that's hurting? There are three different possible culprits for the source of headache pain: the delicate tracery of nerves that covers your scalp; nerves in the face, mouth and throat; and the muscles and blood vessels that cradle and nourish the brain. Once nerve endings in any of these areas are triggered, they send out a pain signal to the brain, and you end up with a headache.

Have you ever wondered what causes a headache? Is it possible to avoid them, or at least reduce their frequency? There are actually several different types of headaches, and each type has its own list of possible causes and treatments. In this book, we will look at the different kinds of headaches and at specialized treatment options available to help make the pain go away. Finally, we will also look at simple lifestyle changes that can keep headaches from starting in the first place.

Nobody deserves to be in pain all the time. Headaches may be among the most common of human afflictions, but they can also be one of the most crippling. For example, the World Health Organization ranked migraines as the 19th most common cause of disability. People who have frequent, severe headaches often find their pain interferes with both work and play.

Primary vs. Secondary Types of Headaches

The modern medical establishment recognizes a variety of different types of headache pain. However, before we look at the different kinds of headache, there are two main categories of headache pain that you should be aware of.

- Primary Headaches - These are the headaches most of us experience on a day-to-day basis. They are called primary headaches because the pain is not a symptom of another physical disorder. Ironically, they are often called "benign" headaches, although headache sufferers would classify them as anything but benign.

- Secondary Headaches - This category of headache includes any headache that is the symptom of another physical disease or disorder. Secondary headaches can be caused by such frightening diseases as aneurysms, blood clots, infections, tumors or a high fever, as well as others.

Secondary headaches require the immediate attention of a doctor in order to treat the condition that is causing the headache. Some of the disorders can be life-threatening if left unattended. So, please see a doctor if you experience anything similar to the following: headaches accompanied by neurological changes such as weakness, inability to talk, or loss of consciousness; headache pain that becomes progressively worse and is the worst headache you've ever experienced; pain that strikes like lightning and is extremely severe; or if you are having to resort to medication on a daily basis.

Types of Primary Headaches

There are several different systems of headache classification as well. However, it is now generally agreed that the most useful or widely accepted system of classifying headaches is that used by the International Headache Society, so it is with the IHS system of headache classification that we will begin.

The earliest classification system which resembles those that are used nowadays was formulated in England by Thomas Willis is 1672.

Nowadays, the mantle of classifying headaches has been taken over by the International Headache Society who published the first edition of the International Classification of Headache Disorders (ICHD) in 1988, with the revised second edition appearing in 2004.

As this system of classifying headaches is accepted by the World Health Organization, it is also one that is most commonly used by medical professionals all over the world as well. The ICHD contains explicit diagnostic criteria that can be applied to various different types of headaches and uses a numerical code to classify the various different types of attack.

At the top of the classification system, there are four different types of headaches that are grouped together under the 'primary headaches' category. These are:

• Tension type headache (TTH);

• Migraine;

• Trigeminal autonomic cephalalgias (TAC) and cluster headaches;

• Other primary headaches including hemicrania continua and new daily persistent headache (NDPH).

Following these four primary types of headaches, there are 14 additional secondary headaches, the majority of which are conditions where the pain in the head is directly accountable to some other form of difficult to your problem. For example, headaches that result from head injury, those that are caused by an infection or by the administration or withdrawal of a particular substance or medication would all be included as secondary headaches.

The headaches that are classified as being primary are conditions where the headache concerned is not caused by any other immediately recognizable condition.

Chapter 2- Signs and Symptoms of Tension Type Headaches

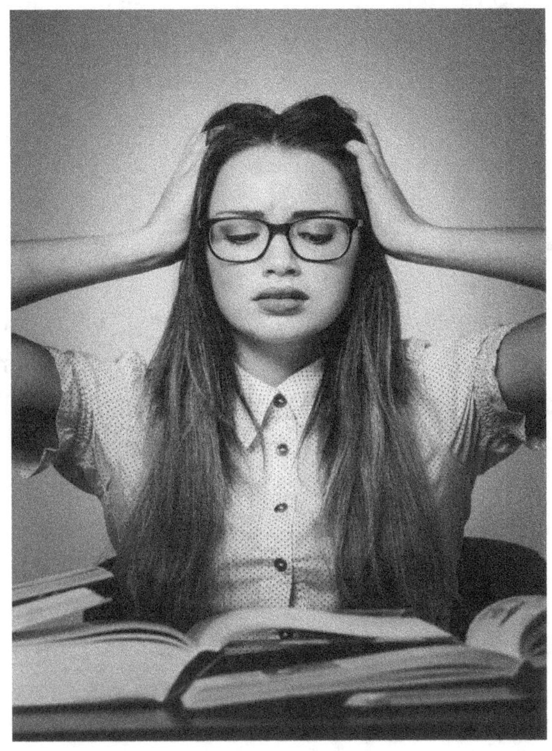

The most common type of headache is tension headaches. Approximately 90% of headaches fall into this category. People with this type of headache typically feel like they have a rubber band wrapped too tightly around their head. The level of pain can vary from mild to fairly severe - in the worst form, pain spreads from the head and covers the shoulders, neck and upper back. Other unpleasant symptoms may also be present. For example, your scalp, neck and shoulder may be sore and painful to touch. You may also feel extremely tired and easily irritated, and may have to struggle to concentrate. Trouble sleeping and a diminished appetite are also common symptoms.

Depending on how often you experience them, tension headaches can be broken down into 3 different classifications. Episodic headaches are usually sporadic and occur less than once a month. Frequent tension headaches happen 1-5 times in a given month. The most frequent type of tension headache is classified as chronic. These can occur 15 or more days per month, which means that sufferers of this type of headache are in pain for at least half of their waking hours.

What Causes a Tension Headache?

As far as the biomechanical mechanisms that make you feel pain are concerned, there are two schools of thought. The first school of thought states that tension headaches are primarily caused by…tension. This theory holds that such factors as stress and anxiety cause muscles in your face, neck and scalp to tense up, causing your headache. However, some researchers today believe that tension headaches don't come from muscle tension at all, but rather from imbalances in brain chemicals and neurotransmitters.

For example, researchers are now able to use special machine called an electromyogram to measure muscle contractions, and they have not found a pattern of increased muscle tension that is specific to tension headaches. People with tension headaches are found to be tense, but not any more or less tense than people with migraines. Additionally, they show alterations in the levels of two very important types of brain chemical: serotonins and endorphins.

Serotonin helps the brain control mood, sleep and appetite, and serotonin imbalances can also cause clinical depression. Endorphins are the body's natural painkillers. Changes in the levels of these chemicals interfere with the body's ability to control pain, and are found in people with both tension headaches and migraines.

No one is sure what causes these changes in brain chemicals. The only thing researchers are certain of right now is that there is a connection between altered levels of these neurotransmitters and various types of headache. However, muscle tension may still be a major contributing factor to tension headache.

What Triggers Tension Type Headaches?

Whatever the precise mechanism is that produces the headache, tension headaches are known to have a variety of different "triggers." Exposure to any one of these triggers can lead to a headache, but different people are sensitive to different "triggers." Here is a list of possible triggers - as you read it, think about the headaches you experience and see if any of these triggers apply to you:

- Stress, depression or anxiety - Heightened emotions, whether they are caused by emotional disorders such as clinical depression or simply from stressful life situations, can trigger headaches in susceptible individuals.

- Lack of sleep, fatigue or overexertion - anything that causes extreme exhaustion can also make you more susceptible to a headache.

- Hunger - Skipping meals or eating at irregular hours gives some people a nasty headache!

- Bad posture - Day-to-day poor posture or any activity that has you holding your head or neck in an awkward or uncomfortable position for a long time will contribute to a headache.

- Eye strain - Staring at a computer screen for too long or reading in poor light leads to headaches for some people.

• Not getting enough exercise

• Excessive smoking, alcohol or caffeine use

• Arthritis and TMD - Both arthritis of the neck and TMD, a disorder that causes excessive jaw clenching, can trigger tension headaches.

• Colds, sinus infections, and nasal congestion - Anyone who's ever had a bad cold can attest to this trigger.

• Overuse of over-the-counter pain relievers can cause a "rebound headache."

CHAPTER 3- SYMPTOMS AND CAUSES OF MIGRAINES

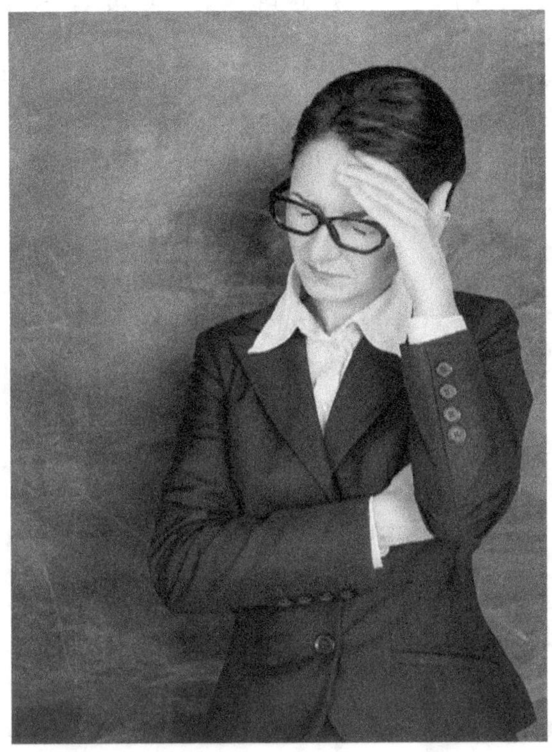

The second type of headache we will discuss is the dreaded migraine. Up to 17% of women and 6% percent of men are believed to have experienced a migraine, and all of you that have had that misfortune know firsthand exactly how disabling migraines can be. A migraine is more than simply a headache. To start with, the pain is usually extremely intense - it can appear either on both sides of the head or be confined to just one side, but it almost always makes your head pulse and throb in agony. The pain often seems to reach a crescendo due to exposure to light or sound, which can effectively make participating in normal daily activities impossible. Additionally, migraine pain usually intensifies in response to physical exertion, often including getting up out of bed.

Another unusual symptom that distinguishes a migraine from other types of headaches is called aura. Aura symptoms can include changes in vision and perception, including a haze around lights, seeing flashes or "stars" in your field of vision, blind spots, and a tingling sensation in arms and legs, almost as if one side of your body has gone to sleep. These strange symptoms usually precede an impending migraine attack, giving you approximately a half hour to go find a dark room to hide in. However, not all migraine sufferers experience aura.

Even if you don't experience aura symptoms, some migraine sufferers will notice changes in mood and energy levels up to a day or so before the migraine strikes. These are known as premonition symptoms, and can include feeling irrationally grumpy, sad or fatigued. However, some people's premonition symptoms are the exact opposite - they report feeling extremely happy and energetic. Other premonition symptoms include being constantly thirsty or craving sweets.

What Causes Migraines?

As is the case with many common medical problems, doctors and scientists are not completely certain about what causes a migraine. Here is a list of what we know so far about the mechanism that produces migraines:

- Migraines are a type of vascular headache, which means that they are thought to be the result of an abnormality in the system of veins and arteries that provides blood to the brain. Basically, these blood vessels widen more than they should, causing pain.

- Migraine victims also suffer from an imbalance of certain brain chemicals, similar to tension headache sufferers.

- People who have recurrent migraines experience a thickening of a region of the brain called the somatosensory cortex, which helps the brain process sensations. However, researchers are not sure yet if this thickening is a potential cause of migraine or an aftereffect.

- The tendency to develop migraines is probably genetic. For example, some studies have found that a child with just one migraine-suffering parent has a 50% chance of also suffering migraine attacks.

Taking all of the knowledge we now have into account, scientists have developed the following theory to explain what causes a migraine. According to this hypothesis, migraine sufferers have a nervous system that overreacts to certain stimuli, called triggers. When someone who is genetically predisposed to experience migraines is exposed to one of their migraine triggers, the unlucky person's nervous system sends out a signal which causes the arteries that supply the brain to spasm.

This spasm causes crucial blood vessels to narrow, which means the brain does not get as much blood as it should. Due to the narrow arteries, platelets in the blood begin to stick together. The action of the platelets causes the brain to release stores of serotonin, which narrows the arteries even more.

By this time, the brain has become increasingly deprived of oxygen, which may explain the aura symptoms described above. In order to re-supply it with fresh, oxygen-rich blood, some arteries inside the brain expand to allow more blood to flow through. Other blood vessels begin to expand as well, until finally the arteries in the scalp and the neck widen also.

Unfortunately, these blood vessels end up over-expanding and become too wide instead of too narrow. This causes the release of chemicals in your body that are associated with pain, inflammation and swelling. The body's response to the release of these chemicals combined with the over-expanded blood vessels in your head is what creates the excruciating pain of a migraine.

Migraines are an extremely crippling form of headache, often making normal life impossible. In fact, the World Health Organization data from 2004 showed that Migraines are one of the top twenty causes of disability. The frequency of headaches can vary from just once a year to almost daily. Once a headache starts, the attack can last anywhere from 4 hours to 6 days before it subsides.

What Triggers Migraines?

Like the triggers for tension headaches, triggers for migraines can vary from person to person, and some people are sensitive to some triggers and not others. Here is a list of possible triggers for migraines:

- Stress, anxiety and depression - Although migraines are by no means a psychosomatic illness, heightened emotional states and stress can be a trigger for some migraine-prone individuals.

- Foods containing tyramine - Tyramine is a substance that causes blood vessels to narrow, possibly setting off the chain reaction described above. Foods that contain tyramine include chocolate, aged cheese, yogurt, nuts, red wine, and processed meats such as summer sausage, bologna and lunch meats.

- Foods containing MSG - Foods such as Chinese food and many processed foods are high in this chemical, and may trigger migraines in some people.

- Lack of sleep or too much sleep - Any change in your normal sleep routine may trigger a migraine.

- Caffeine - Caffeine can trigger migraines in people who are sensitive to it.

- Skipping meals

- Changes in the weather - For some people, something as simple and natural as the changing of the seasons or a storm moving through may set off a migraine.

- Hormonal changes - In women, any event that causes hormone levels to fluctuate can also trigger a migraine. This includes menstruation, menopause, pregnancy, and possibly taking birth control pills.

- Sensory Overload - Bright lights or strong smells are also possible migraine triggers.

- Overexertion - This can include too much exercise, and for some extremely unfortunate individuals, too much sex.

Migraine triggers vary from person to person, so the list above describes the most common triggers. However, it is far from exhaustive. If you suffer from migraines and nothing on this list rings a bell, don't worry.

Chapter 4- Understanding Cluster Headaches

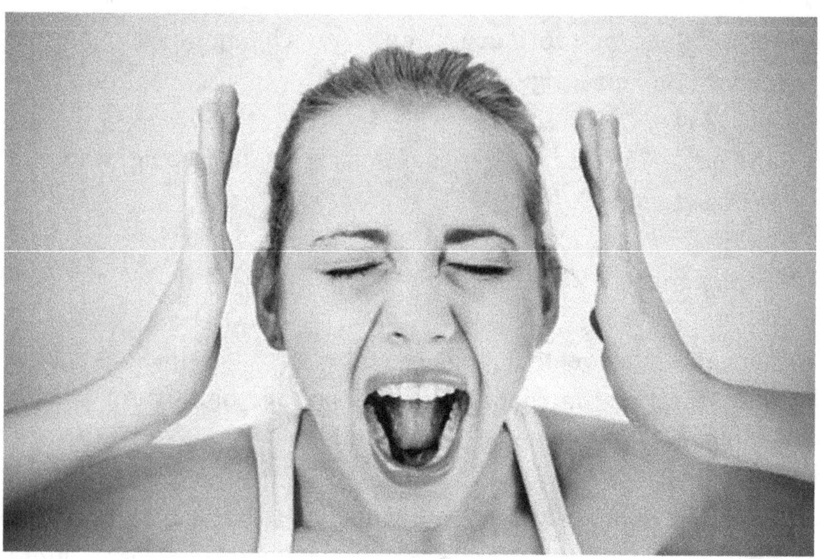

A cluster headache is one of the most excruciating kinds of headache, surpassing even the pain of an average migraine in intensity. It is generally described as a sharp, stabbing type of pain that lacks the throbbing, pulsating quality of a migraine. Cluster headache attacks happen extremely fast - one minute the person feels perfectly normal, the next minute like they are being stabbed through the eye. Generally, the pain is located on just one side of the head.

Cluster headaches often occur in tandem with other symptoms, which are usually limited to the side of the face that the pain is on. For example, the victim's pupils may shrink in size, one eye may suddenly start overflowing with tears or the eyelid may start drooping, and the affected side of the face may swell or turn red.

The defining feature of a cluster headache is that the attacks are experienced in waves or cycles, also called clusters. Clusters can last from 2 days to a couple of weeks. During the cluster period, attacks usually occur at least once per day, although they can occur more often. Many times, cluster attack victims are jerked out of a sound sleep by a severe headache. The length of each individual headache is relatively short, however; anywhere from a half hour to an hour and a half.

After the cluster period ends, the victim may experience a pain-free period of remission, when the headaches do not occur. People who experience cluster periods followed by remission have what is known as episodic cluster headache. Other people have chronic cluster headache, with no remission period between cycles.

What Causes Cluster Headaches?

Cluster headaches are even more shrouded in mystery than tension headaches and migraines. Nobody is quite sure what causes these painful attacks, and the scientific hypotheses we have so far are not very detailed. For example, some researchers believe that cluster headaches are caused by a disruption in the nerve system that carries sensations from your head to your brain. This system of nerves is called the trigeminal system.

Other doctors believe that the pain starts with blood vessels buried deep in your head, such as the arteries that run through your sinuses. The hypothalamus, the control center for the body's circadian rhythms or "biological clock," is probably involved as well. That would explain why cluster attacks occur in such a regular pattern.

What Triggers Cluster Headaches?

Unlike migraines and tension headaches, cluster headaches lack a set of easily definable triggers. However, there are a few events that seem to bring on attacks:

• Changing seasons - for some people, cluster headaches are associated with a particular season of the year. These people may suffer a cluster attack during the same time each year (for example, every winter or every fall). Other people are particularly prone to cluster attacks after the solstices, the longest and shortest days of the year.

• Alcohol - Alcohol is not known to start off a cluster of attacks. But, once the cluster starts, even a small amount of alcohol can bring on a headache.

Cluster headaches affect 1 in every 1,000 people. They are the rarest type of primary headache, and affect men more frequently than women. However, for cluster headache sufferers, the pain is a serious and debilitating affliction. Some people have even been known to attempt suicide during an attack due to the severity of the pain.

CHAPTER 5- OTHER TYPES OF HEADACHES NOT ASSOCIATED WITH MEDICAL CONDITIONS

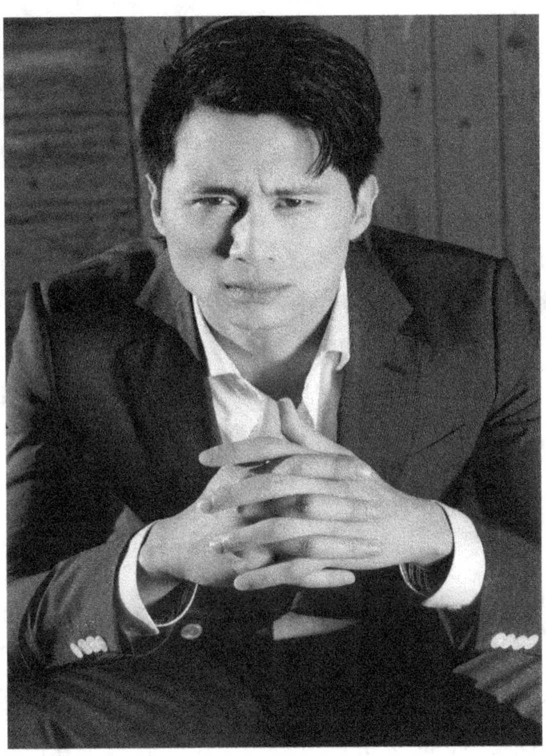

There are a few other forms of headache that are categorized as being primary conditions because they are not caused by or associated with other medical conditions.

• Hemicrania Continua

Hemicrania continua is a persistent unilateral headache that is most commonly unremitting. According to the International Headache Society system of classification, for Hemicrania continua to be diagnosed, the sufferer has to have been blighted by their headache for a period of at least three months whilst demonstrating all of the following symptoms:

• There must be persistent unilateral pain which does not shift;

• The pain must be continuous and daily, without remission and

• The pain should usually be of moderate intensity, although there may be periods when the pain level increases markedly.

In addition to these three criteria and the requirement that the headache should have lasted for at least three months, your doctor would expect to see related eye or nose problems as well, such as crying or suffering from nasal congestion.

Very occasionally, there have been reports of occasional examples where remission does happen where Hemicrania is still diagnosed because in all other respects, the sufferer's headache problem exactly matches all other requirements for Hemicrania continua.

• New Daily Persistent Headache

This is a condition which has only recently been recognized as a distinct type of primary headache by the International Headache Society, with the criteria for recognizing the condition being laid down in the second ICHD in 2004.

These first criteria for recognizing a new daily persistent headache is that it is a headache that the patient has been suffering from for at least three months, and that it satisfies the following requirements as well:

• The pain must be felt daily and must be unremitting;

• It must demonstrate at least of the four following characteristics;

1. The pain must be bilateral;

2. The feeling of the pain must be of pressing or tightening, not pulsing or throbbing;

3. The pain must be mild to moderate and

4. It should not be aggravated by normal daily physical activity such as walking or climbing the stairs;

• The headache should also demonstrate both of the following qualities as well;

1. The patient must not be suffering more than one of phonophobia (sensitivity to noise) or photophobia (light) or mild nausea and

2. There should be no serious nausea or vomiting either.

Because this particular form of headache exhibits some of the characteristics of tension type headaches and some of the characteristics of migraine, it is a condition that is not particularly easy to diagnose.

Furthermore, because other far more serious conditions such as a spontaneous cerebrospinal leak can mimic some of the indicators of this particular form of headache, it is necessary for doctors to run many other tests such as an MRI scan to rule these more serious potential problems out before arriving at diagnosis.

In addition, many doctors might also consider taking a lumbar puncture sample as well to rule out an infection before finally arriving at a diagnosis of new daily persistent headache.

Chapter 6- Headache Treatments per Type

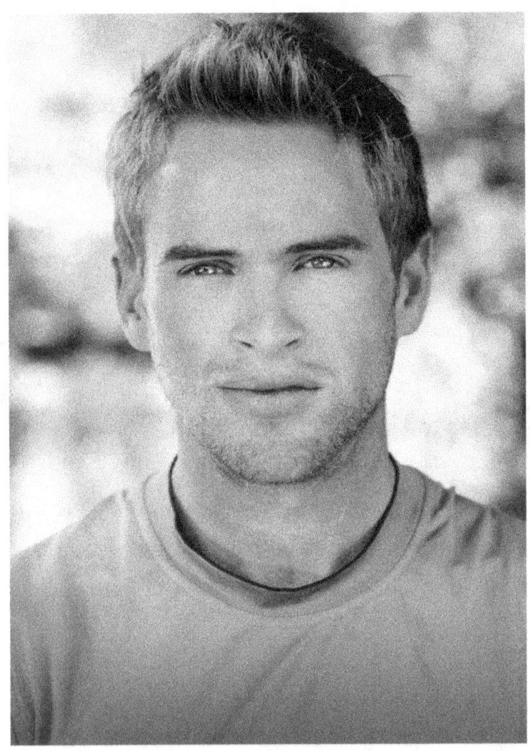

If you are amongst the fortunate majority who only suffer headaches every so often, you will probably have gathered by now that for those who are less fortunate that suffer headaches on a regular or persistent basis, seeking medical attention is often necessary.

Although irregular headache sufferers would probably never consider doing anything more than taking an over-the-counter painkiller to get rid of their headache, for those who suffer the worst ravages of primary headaches, self-medicating with painkillers in this way is not always a viable option.

Consequently, I am going to consider and highlight many of the medical treatments that your doctor may prescribe if you are a persistent or regular headache sufferer whilst also pointing out some of the potential side-effects of those drugs that you should be aware of.

For Tension Type Headaches

If you are a person who only suffers headaches every now and then, then you are more than likely an episodic tension type headache sufferer.

In this case, most sufferers are likely to turn to an over-the-counter analgesic painkiller to treat their condition.

For chronic tension type headache sufferers, there are many different types of drugs prescribed which will be known by a wide variety of brand names. Some of the most commonly prescribed drugs are as follows:

• Amitriptyline

This drug goes under a huge range of different brand names. And although it was originally used as an antidepressant, it is nowadays often prescribed for people who suffer chronic tension type headaches or migraine, albeit in relatively small doses.

Some of the less pleasant side-effects suffered by some users are weight gain, nausea, constipation, dizziness, dry mouth, blurred vision and insomnia. In more serious cases, the drug has been seen to cause hypotension, psychosis, arrhythmias, heart blockage and depression.

• Mirtazapine

Mirtazapine (known as Remeron in the USA, Canada, Australia and South Africa but as Zispin or Zispin Soltab in the UK and Ireland) is a psychoactive drug that is primarily used as an antidepressant.

In addition to being used as an antidepressant, it has also been found to be effective in the treatment of migraine and chronic tension type headaches, although once again, it is a drug with a long list of potential adverse side-effects attached to it.

The common side-effects include blurred vision, dizziness, sedation, increased appetite and accompanying weight gain, shallow breathing or hypoventilation, malaise, decrease body temperature, restless leg syndrome and many, many more.

More seriously, side effects may include convulsions or seizures, excessive water retention and edemas, nausea and vomiting, diarrhea, sexual dysfunction and depression or anxiety that can in the most serious cases border on suicidal behavior.

In addition, the drug has also caused mild to moderate psychedelic experiences and effects in some patients, although whether everyone would necessarily agree that this is an adverse side-effect is open to debate!

• Sodium valproate

Some doctors may consider using sodium valproate as a prophylaxis, that is, a drug that is designed to prevent chronic tension type headaches rather than get rid of them.

The main use of sodium valproate is as an antiepileptic drug, with the main downside of this particular drug being that the chances of a baby being born with a birth defect to anyone taking this particular drug are somewhere between two and five times higher than they are with other antiepileptic drugs.

Furthermore, there is some evidence that children born to a mother who is taking a valproate drug have a significantly higher chance of suffering autism as well according to a study carried out in 2005 by the Autism Association of America.

For Migraines

Both of the main prescription drugs that your doctor is likely to prescribe for dealing with chronic tension type headaches are also often prescribed for combating the worst effects of migraine as well.

Some doctors may also consider prescribing sodium valproate as well as a prophylactic to prevent the onset of migraine headaches before they start.

There are however some different forms of treatments that might be prescribed to deal with migraine headaches, with the first line of attack generally being over-the-counter analgesics like aspirin, Tylenol and paracetamol (acetaminophen in North America). If the individual suffering from a migraine headache is fortunate enough for it to be only a mild attack, such analgesics will probably be strong enough to deal with the problem, although whether you want to take analgesics is another matter entirely (for reasons highlighted later).

Sometimes these analgesics will be taken or rendered entirely on their own whereas at other times, it might be prescribed or taken in combination with other substances such as caffeine. Whilst migraine sufferers are generally advised to limit their caffeine intake, it does seem that combining analgesics with caffeine enhances the effectiveness of the drug (and caffeine is itself recognized as an over-the-counter drug by the FDA).

As suggested earlier, migraine headaches are often accompanied by nausea and/or vomiting, so it is not uncommon for the analgesics rendered to be combined with antiemetic drugs as well.

For migraines that do not respond to over-the-counter drugs or other analgesics, your doctor may prescribe a serotonin specific reuptake inhibitors (SSRI) which are effective in getting rid of mild-to-moderate migraine headaches that do not respond to analgesics or other first-line drug defenses.

Although SSRIs are not approved by the FDA for the treatment of migraine headaches, tests and trials have indicated that they can help in certain circumstances.

Technically speaking, the primary usage of SSRIs is as an antidepressant drug and once again, there is a long list of potential adverse side-effects which you might suffer if you choose to take one of these drugs to deal with your migraine problem.

These side-effects include apathy, nausea and vomiting, drowsiness, dizziness, changes in appetite and sleep patterns, tremors and weight loss or weight gain.

Most of these side-effects are felt soon after starting to take the drugs as your body gets used to them and many of them will pass.

However, it is also known for SSRIs to cause far more serious side-effects, with some patients reporting sexual problems and cardiovascular side-effects. Furthermore, because they are anti-depressant drugs, SSRIs can create a degree of dependency in any patient who takes them for anything other than the shortest period of time.

Other forms of treatment that might be used as a way of dealing with migraine headaches include ergot alkaloids which though effective for aborting migraine headaches once they have started come with their own attendant panoply of potential side-effects.

For example, ergotism is a condition where the cumulative effects of taking ergot alkaloid-based medicines or drugs builds up over time and gradually poisons your body.

A proprietary drug like Cafergot probably works because both caffeine and ergot work as vasoconstrictors meaning that they narrow the blood vessels which helps to regulate the blood supply. This in turn should help reduce the severity of the migraine attack.

However, drugs like Cafergot are not all that easy to obtain in the USA or the UK and they do have potential side-effects such as causing numbness in your toes and fingers, angina pectoris, blurred vision and dizziness. These are all potential side-effects which are caused by the general vasoconstriction which happens all over your body, not just in your brain.

In addition to all of these drugs that your doctor may prescribe for you to help you get rid of your migraine headache, they may also suggest a wide range of drugs which you would take to prevent the initial onset of migraine before you suffered the attack.

There are many drugs that might be offered such as beta-blockers, anticonvulsants and antidepressants. All of these drugs will have potential adverse side-effects attached to them depending upon the particular drug being prescribed.

Anne Higgins
OTC Drugs and Their Side Effects

Perhaps you might think that because they are openly sold in pharmacies and drug stores with government approval that all over-the-counter analgesics must be safe, but this is an assumption that you should not allow yourself to make. Despite the fact that drugs sold in most western countries have to be government approved, the fact that they are should never be taken as proving that they are completely safe because even the most common or garden analgesics and do have potential side-effects.

For example, although it has been on open sale for more than 100 years, the humble aspirin does have acknowledged adverse side-effects in some people including stomach ulcers and gastrointestinal bleeding. Large doses of salicylate (which is a metabolite of aspirin) have been shown to cause tinnitus in rats, and it is not at all uncommon for people who take aspirin reasonably regularly to develop swelling and hives.

In a worst case scenario, it is also known that aspirin can cause a little-known condition known as Reyes Syndrome in children, which can cause serious damage to the brain and liver and might ultimately prove fatal.

If you are taking paracetamol (acetaminophen), there is a long list of possible side effects attached to the drug even though it is highly effective as a painkiller, especially when paired with other painkillers such as codeine as it often is in over-the-counter medicines.

Nevertheless, taken in large doses, paracetamol can cause liver failure and ultimately death – it is the number-one cause of acute liver failure in both the USA and the UK – but even at regular dosage levels, the same results can occur in some unfortunate people.

Furthermore, excessive use of paracetamol might cause serious damage to other internal organs, whilst some studies have indicated that the drug can cause internal bleeding in even relatively small dosages too.

The bottom line is, even apparently safe and benign over-the-counter analgesics are not necessarily as safe as you might imagine them to be with plenty of nasty potential side-effects.

As suggested, this might give you cause to re-consider whether using chemical-based analgesics is such a good idea after all.

Medical Treatments Applicable to All Types of Headaches

1. Butalbital combinations

Butalbital is a sedative that is often combined with analgesics such as aspirin or acetametaphin, and sometimes caffeine or codeine. It is used for migraines and severe tension headaches.

- These combinations are used infrequently due to side effects.

- Side effects can include rebound headaches and withdrawal symptoms.

2. Oxygen Inhalation Treatment

Oxygen inhalation is used as a medical treatment for cluster headaches. Pure oxygen is inhaled through a mask for up to 10-15 minutes. This often leads to a rapid release from the grasp of a cluster headache - up to 80% of patients reported relief in trials.

3. Midrin

Midrin combines a blood vessel constrictor, an analgesic and a light sedative into one package. It is effective for both migraine and tension headaches.

- Midrin is taken orally.

- Possible side effects include dizziness, drowsiness, rash, and withdrawal symptoms when trying to stop using the drug.

As you can see, there are many different drug regimens that can be used to help treat your headaches. However, please remember that only a doctor can tell you if these medications are right for you or not.

4. Triptans

Triptans are a class of drugs prescribed specifically for migraines and cluster headaches, although they can also be used by people affected by both chronic migraines and chronic tension headaches. In addition to relieving headache pain, they can also help with nausea, vomiting, and other symptoms associated with migraines.

- Triptans work by causing the over-dilated blood vessels in your brain to shrink back to normal size, normalizing the flow of blood in the brain.

- They also prevent the release of brain chemicals that contribute to inflammation and pain.

- Triptans can stop a migraine once it starts. Statistically speaking, they successfully stop 80% of migraine attacks.

- These drugs come in 3 forms: oral, injectable and a nose spray. The injections and the nose spray are the fastest-acting.

- Potential side effects can include body aches, tiredness, dry mouth, tingling sensations, weakness and throwing up.

- Rare, but more serious side effects can include a stroke or a heart attack. So, do not pass go and go directly to the nearest emergency room if you feel chest pain or pressure, get dizzy or have trouble breathing after taking triptans.

- Some common triptan brand names include Imetrix, Maxalt, Amerge, Zomig, Axert, Frova, and Relpax.

Chapter 7- Natural Remedies to Consider

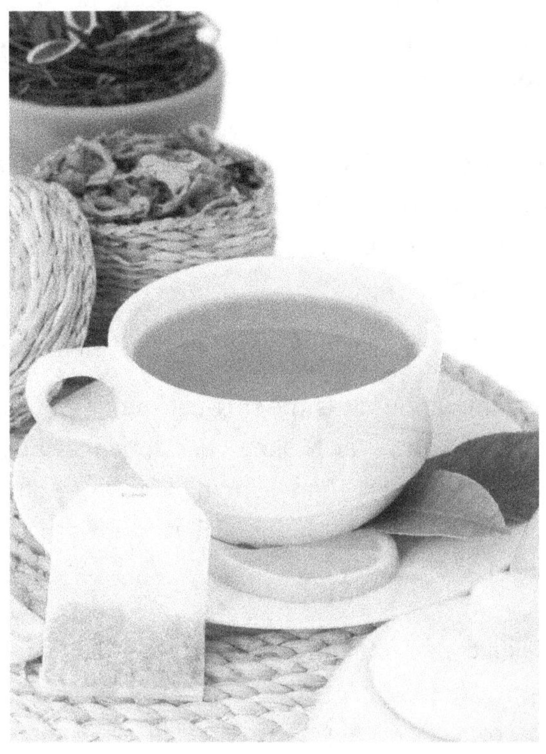

For people who just don't want to use drugs or can't handle the side effects, there are also natural remedies available. These have the advantage of being as effective as drug therapy in some cases, and they are often cheaper than drugs and have fewer side effects. Here is a look at some popular non-drug approaches to treating headaches.

Herbal Remedies

Long before Western medicine showed up on the scene, people used plants to treat themselves for various ailments. Many of these herbal remedies are surprisingly effective, having been shown to work over centuries of use. In many cases, their effectiveness is now being proven to the Western world in scientific studies. Some of the herbs commonly used to treat headaches include:

- Feverfew - This herb is a small relative of the sunflower that looks much like a miniature daisy. It has been used as an anti-inflammatory for centuries in traditional medicine. Feverfew has been shown in several studies to be effective in both prevention and treatment of migraines. To use feverfew to stop a migraine, take 100-300 mg of the herb. If you are allergic to yarrow, chamomile, or ragweed, please avoid feverfew because you may be allergic to it, also.

- Willow Bark - Willow bark has been used for centuries to treat pain and inflammation - it is the original source of aspirin, and is equally effective. However, willow bark appears to be less likely to upset your stomach than aspirin. Since aspirin can cause Reye's syndrome in children under 16, it is advised to also avoid giving willow bark to them.

- Valerian, skullcap, and lemon balm - Used separately or in combination, these herbs possess both sedative and anti-spasmodic properties. They can help relax you and help to de-constrict your arteries, restoring proper blood flow to your brain. These herbs are available in the form of capsules, tea and tinctures. These are effective in tension headaches and possibly for migraines.

- Cayenne - A cayenne pepper solution can be used as a nose spray to help relieve a cluster headache. However, this treatment can cause pain and a burning sensation in the nose. Talk to a naturopath or doctor to find a suitable preparation.

- Ginger - Ginger may be effective in treating migraine headaches. There was a case study where a woman who suffered from chronic migraines began taking ginger at the first sign of aura and was able to head off her headache. Ginger has anti-inflammatory properties and is known to help fight off nausea. There currently have not been any standardized experiments done on ginger, but to see if it works for you, take 500 to 600 milligrams of powdered ginger in water.

- Ginkgo Biloba - Although this herb is better-known as a memory enhancer, it can also help stop migraine pain. Ginkgo widens blood vessels and helps improve circulation, keeping a normal amount of blood and oxygen flowing to the brain.

- Coffee - Coffee contains caffeine, which has been shown effective in treating headaches. However, be aware that many over-the-counter drugs for headaches, such as Excedrin, also contain caffeine.

Aromatherapy

People have always taken great pleasure in the scent of certain plants and herbs. However, aromatherapy is about more than perfume. Aromatherapy harnesses the power of essential plant oils and fragrances to enhance health and well-being.

Don't be fooled by "aromatherapy" products that contain synthetic fragrance oils instead of real essential oils. To get the benefits, you need to inhale the volatile compounds from the plant itself, compounds found only in real essential oils.

For aromatherapy, you can take a warm bath with essential oils in the bathwater, apply just a drop or two of skin-safe oil to your skin, or place a few drops in a bowl of hot water and inhale the steam. Most essential oils should not be applied to your skin at full strength. Instead, you should dilute to a 2% concentration using a carrier oil to avoid skin irritation.

Here are some essential oils commonly used in the treatment of headaches:

- Peppermint - Stimulates blood flow and has a pain-relieving effect that may be as strong as acetaminophen. Inhale vapors, or apply a drop to your temples.

- Sandalwood - Applied in a paste made with clay to the temples. This is a popular remedy from India.

- Lavender - Lavender is a sedative that also relieves pain. This oil can safely be used "neat," without diluting it in carrier oil.

- Rosemary - Stimulates blood flow and helps relieve pain. Can be combined with lavender oil and rubbed directly on stiff neck muscles to relax them.

- Rose oil - Rose oil massaged onto your face will help lift a headache.

- Frankincense - Frankincense oil can be applied full-strength at the base of the skull.

Biofeedback

The mind-body connection is a potent force that is still little-understood. However, doctors and scientists are learning more and more about this connection, and biofeedback is one result of our increased knowledge. With biofeedback, the patient is taught how to control bodily functions that until recently were thought to be involuntary. For example, heart rate, body temperature, brain activity and muscle tension.

How does biofeedback work? Basically, you are hooked up to a machine that uses sensors to measure the bodily functions you are trying to learn to control. For example, your therapist might hook you up to an electromyogram, which is a machine that measures muscle tension.

The machine lets you know when the tension level in your muscles changes - for example, it may make noise or light up. By learning to sense when your muscles are starting to tense up, you can also learn to control that tension and relax them.

In addition to biofeedback for muscle tension, biofeedback to control body temperature is commonly used for migraines. People that learn how to raise their body temperature report that they are able to control their migraines.

The link between body temperature and pain relief for migraines is that in order for your body temperature to rise, your blood vessels have to get wider. Thus, if you can learn to raise your body temperature, you can learn to control the flow of blood into your brain and cut off the chain reaction that results in a migraine headache.

Acupuncture and Acupressure

Acupuncture is an ancient Chinese science that has been in use for thousands of years. However, it is relatively new to Western culture and is still seen as a form of alternative medicine. Acupuncture uses extremely thin needles (much thinner than a hypodermic needle) that are inserted into specific points on the body.

Cure Headaches Naturally

Acupuncture is based on the concept of an invisible energy system that circulates through our bodies along paths referred to as "meridians." This energy is called "chi." In ancient Chinese medical theory, many illnesses were thought to result when a person's chi was blocked and prevented from circulating properly.

Acupuncture uses needles to stimulate certain pressure points along the meridians, which is believed to correct the flow of chi in the body. Of course, the existence of "chi" is not universally acknowledged in Western medicine, and many doctors either question acupuncture's effectiveness or look for other explanations for it. However it works, many studies have shown that acupuncture is able to help people with a variety of conditions, including headaches.

Acupressure is a type of massage therapy that is based on the principles of acupuncture. Basically, the same pressure points are stimulated, but instead of using needles, strong pressure is applied by the therapists' fingers. This treatment is appropriate for people who want to try acupuncture but are terrified of needles.

Unlike acupuncture, which must be practiced by an acupuncturist, acupressure can be used at home. This makes it extremely convenient for treating headaches as they occur.

To try acupressure on yourself, you can very firmly massage the webbed area in between your thumb and forefinger, at the point where the finger bone and thumb bone meet and form a "V." This is considered one of the best pressure points for a headache, and it's also by far the easiest to reach on your own. You can also try massaging the points on each side of the neck vertebrae, right where the muscles of your neck meet your skull.

Homeopathy

Homeopathy is a system of medicine developed by Samuel Hahnemann, a German doctor, in the late 18th century. Homeopathic remedies follow the basic principles he laid out, namely, "like cures like" and the "law of infinitesimals."

The principle of "like cures like" basically states that a homeopathic remedy is chosen based on the symptoms it would produce if taken in large quantities in a healthy person. Homeopathic practitioners look for a substance that produces similar systems to what the patient is suffering. Since "like cures like," that substance will become the remedy.

The "law of infinitesimals" states that only very small dosages of the substance are necessary. These highly diluted doses prompt the body to react with a natural healing response that also corrects the original ailment.

There are various types of homeopathic remedies, each for a specific set of headache symptoms. The following list contains only a few examples. To find the correct remedy for your specific headache, it is recommended that you visit a licensed homeopath.

- Belladonna - Highly diluted solutions of belladonna are given when the patient experiences the following symptoms: extremely intense, stabbing pains on one side of the head, change in pupil size, flushing on one side of the face - basically, all the symptoms of a classic cluster headache.

- Natrum muriaticum - This substance is recommended for throbbing headaches accompanied by disturbances of vision, symptoms that seem to indicate a migraine.

- Gelsemium is recommended as a homeopathic remedy for tension headaches, characterized by the feeling of having a rubber band drawn too tightly around the head.

Mind over Matter

Another drug-free method of treating headaches is to practice relaxation techniques to help relax your muscles and clear your mind of stress. Some people find techniques such as meditation and creative visualization to be quite helpful in stopping a headache.

Meditation

Meditation is one relaxation technique that has been studied for migraines. In the study, participants who meditated reported experiencing fewer migraines than people who did not meditate.

Many religions practice some form of meditation, so there are many different types of meditation. However, they all share a common goal: to help the participant learn to focus their attention entirely in the present moment. By living life one moment at a time, much of the stress that triggers headaches can be avoided or diminished.

Although meditation can be part of religious practice for some people, it certainly does not have to be. Many people practice meditation simply to gain greater mental discipline and better control over their thoughts, or to relieve stress.

Visualization and Guided Imagery

Visualization and guided imagery are powerful relaxation techniques. Like meditation, they rely on harnessing the power of the mind to heal the body. However, the difference between meditation and using guided imagery is that meditation is about clearing your mind completely. With guided imagery, on the other hand, instead of clearing your mind, you focus on a set of healing images.

For example, some people visualize standing in front of a giant medicine cabinet, choosing a bottle from the cabinet, and taking a pill. The idea is that simply imagining taking a headache pill that you know will work causes the body to behave as if under the influence of the imaginary medication. Thus, your headache goes away.

Another sample guided imagery technique is to imagine your headache as a ball of red light that fills up the inside of your skull. If your head is pounding, imagine the light pulsing in time with your pain.

Now, imagine that your hands are producing a gentle azure light, like starlight. Bring your hands up to your head, placing them wherever the pain is most intense. Imagine the cool starlight from your hands chasing away the hot red light in your head, and you should feel your pain diminish along with the red light.

Hot and Cold Therapy

Using heat and cold to relieve pain is another natural method of treating a headache. For example, an ice cold compress applied to the temples relieves headache pain for some people. When the headache is accompanied by pain in the neck area, a warm compress will relax muscles and reduce headache-triggering tension. Alternating hot and cold showers will help increase circulation and may help with migraines.

Chapter 8- Tips to Prevent Headaches

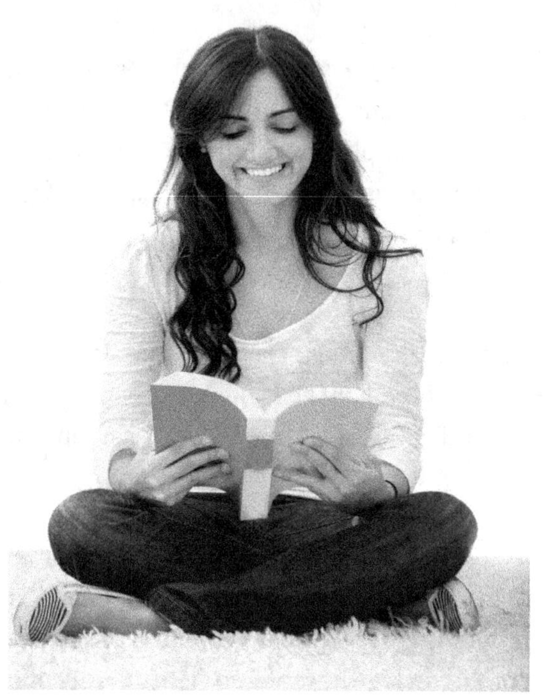

1.Keep a Diary

Keeping a headache diary is perhaps the most important part of any prevention routine. A "headache diary" will allow you to keep track of your headaches and discover what triggers them.

For example, try to remember what you ate or drank the last time you had a headache. What was the weather like? Did anything stressful happen that day? Chances are, you don't remember anymore, even if it was just a few days ago.

A headache diary is crucial because it allows you to write down all of the possible factors that could have triggered your headache.

Then, you can begin looking for patterns until you isolate your own personal headache triggers.

Start by comparing your headache diary entry with the common triggers for the type of headache you are experiencing. If your headaches don't seem to correlate with any of the triggers mentioned in the book, simply start looking for patterns. Look at your entry and for every day that you had a headache, think: What does today have in common with last time I had a headache?

If your headache triggers turn out to be something that's easily avoided, such as a certain type of food, you can consider cutting the trigger out of your life completely.

Some triggers, of course, will be uncontrollable factors like stress, or the weather. While you cannot hope to avoid these types of factors completely, once you realize that they are setting off headaches you can take preventative steps as soon as you are exposed to the trigger.

To help you get started on your diary, here is an example of a sample page:

- Date and Time
- Warning signs/Aura
- Foods eaten today
- Weather
- Stress level, emotional state
- Hours slept last night
- Daily activities leading up to headache
- Duration of headache

Once you understand what causes a headache, it is often much easier to treat and prevent. Hopefully, this book has given you the knowledge you need to manage your headaches and improve your quality of life!

2. Follow the Proper Way to Read

Do not read when you are lying down. The lying down posture is clearly not the best position to read. It is a very common thing for a person to flop down on the bed with a book and read it while lying down. In fact, many people make it a habit to read for a few minutes before going to sleep. Let us say it once and for all; it is not good to read while you are lying down. If you must read, prop up your head with at least two pillows. If you find it impossible to read while you are in bed, the best thing that you can do is prop up your head with a couple of pillows. Pillows give support to your head and neck so that your head is in a partially raised position. This will cause less harm to your eyes and your head in general.

You need a well-lighted room to read. The lighting of your room too is very important. A properly lighted room is what is required if you want to read, do needle work or any other such fine activity. Again too much light is just as bad as a dimly lit room. The source of light must preferably be behind your head. The source of light should not come in front of your eyes but must be behind your head. This is also true in the case of a computer as well. The source of light should be from behind.

Do not hold the book too close to your eyes. This is something that happens when you lay down to read. The book tends to move closer to your eyes than intended. This is something that is bad for your eyes. Your eye muscles have to strain a lot in order to focus on nearer objects. The book should ideally be at the level of your chest. Do not hold it too far away either. Holding the book too far away is just as bad as holding the book too close. Remember to keep it at chest level. Many bookstores have reading stands that will enable you to keep your book position at the right level.

If you find it difficult to read, get your eyes tested by an oculist. If you find yourself squinting or your eyes watering while you read or do any fine work, then you might need glasses. So do not waste time, consult a doctor at the earliest time possible. Faulty vision is a major cause of headaches. Be careful of the print size of the book you are reading. If the print of the book is too faint, or if the font size is too small, just toss away the book. Most libraries have large print versions of books. If this is not available, use a magnifying glass or wear magnifying glasses.

Do not read in moving vehicles. Many people try to read while traveling by car to kill time. However, curves and bumps in the road can cause headaches and even motion sickness. No matter how smooth the road is and no matter how good the shock absorbers of the car are, there is bound to be jerking motions. This will force your eyes to adjust and readjust to the print and this continuous adjustment and readjustment is very bad for your eyes. At the end of the journey you are bound to end up with a headache.

3. Take Breaks from Work

While doing work that requires you to strain your eyes, take breaks every five minutes. This is especially true for jobs like needle work and works involving electronic gadgets. Use an anti-glare screen to cut out the radiation while working on your computer. Radiation is bad for your eyes and an anti-glare screen is the only and the best solution to this.

Another option is to wear glasses that have an anti-glare coating on the lenses. If your job requires long hours in front of the computer, you may want to consider buying a special lamp that clips on the monitor. This lamp reduces the eye-strain caused by staring at the computer screen, and thus reduces headaches.

4. Protect Your Eyes

Never look at the sun directly, especially between 7 am in the morning and 4 pm in the evening. If you will be outside during this time or driving, be sure to shield your eyes in some manner.

While going outdoors during the summer, protect your eyes using sunglasses. Sunglasses are the best protection that you can give your eyes when you go out in the sun. The sun beats down ultra violet and other harmful radiations. Your eyes need protection from these radiations because they can cause serious damage to your eyes if they are directly exposed to them. Below are some tips for choosing sunglasses.

- The sunglasses must cover the region of your eyes completely.

- Sunglasses may be of any color that you like but make sure that they guard your eyes against ultra violet radiations.

- Take care to see that your sunglasses are always clean and free from dust and smudges.

- The best way to choose your sunglasses is to put them on and stare at your face in a mirror. If you can see your eyes in the mirror, then the glasses are not good enough.

- Do not work continuously on your computer for more than half an hour. This in fact is a very relative concept because some people tire faster than other when working on the computer. Computer screens emit radiation, so the less time in front of the computer, the better.

If your eyes give you signs that it has had enough take the cue. But often, after you get used to working on the computer, you start ignoring these signs. The best thing you can do is make it a point to give your eyes a break at least every half hour of working on the computer.

The best rest that you can give your eyes is staring at a distant object. Or you can try massaging your eyes gently. Please remember that your eyes are unlike any other part of your body so you have to take very good care of them. The same holds true when it comes to massaging your eyes as well.

- When you massage your eyes take care to use only the soft balls of your fingers.

- Do not use your fingertips because your nails could give you scratches.

- The best fingers to massage your eyes with are the three middle fingers, which are the fingers between your thumb and the little finger.

- Place the balls of your fingers on your eye brows and gently press down.

- Please remember to be gentle; we are not talking about a major massage therapy here.

- Now let your fingers roll down around your eyes making gentle circling movements.

- The motion should start from the eye brows and end at the corners of the eyes near the nose bridge.

- Repeat this two or three times and you can feel your eye muscles relax.

- It is a good idea to this at least five or six times a day if you are working at something that gives a lot of strain to your eyes.

5.Try Breathing Exercises

Breathing exercises help you breathe better and release the toxins in your brain. The human body takes in a lot of toxic substances, both through the air and through food and drink. Apart from this, various toxins are also released in the body as a result of the various processes that are going on. These toxins have to be released on a continuous basis or else they will accumulate in the body with serious results.

One of the best ways of releasing these toxins is by means of exhaling while breathing. One funny fact is that most of do not breathe properly. Just take a look at the picture like this. With each breath that we take, we take in oxygen. This oxygen is carried by the blood to every cell of the body and every cell must indeed get enough oxygen not just to survive but to remain healthy as well.

So it is imperative that we make an honest attempt to breathe properly. But first of course we have to make sure that we are breathing in unpolluted air. The time best for breathing exercises is early in the morning when the air is comparatively unpolluted. Now what you have to do is this. Again, sit comfortably so that there is no strain to any part of your body. It is not imperative that you close your eyes, but I have always noticed that the exercise works better when the eyes are closed. When you are ready, what you have to do is to breathe in deeply and slowly, and feel the fresh air filling up your lungs until it just can't take any more.

Conjure up images of the air encircling throughout your body and reaching every cell, literally bathing it with oxygen. Of course it doesn't happen that way but the image helps a lot. Then hold your breath for a few seconds and then very slowly exhale letting out all that foul air. Again conjure up an image of all the toxins being released from your body. Every cell has become free of the burden it was carrying. Now pause for a second or two and again breathe in deeply, slowly letting your lungs fill up with all that good, clean, rejuvenating air.

Repeat this exercise at least ten times and take your time for it taking care not to rush through. When you have done that part of the exercise it is time for the second part. Again sit with your eyes closed, but this time, keep one nostril closed with the help of your index finger. It is best to close the right nostril first and that too with your right index finger.

Now breathe in deeply and slowly through your left nostril keeping the right nostril closed. When you have held air for a second or two, release your right nostril and breathe out through it. While you are breathing out conjure up an image of all the toxins being released form your head and the brain especially. And as you breathe in conjure up images of the clean air circulating though out your brain freeing it of all the worries and trouble and lightening it. Repeat this exercise with the other nostril closed and in this way alternate between the nostrils at least ten times. The entire breathing exercise need not take more than ten minutes.

6. Dry Your Hair

Dry your head well after a shower. It is best to use a towel for this. The problem with water is that it can seep in through the scalp of your head and if you leave your head damp, the moisture can seep in result in a headache.

Do not blow dry your hair as far as possible. Dryers are not a very good idea. The heat from the dryer is actually bad for your head. Go easy on driers and if at all you must use a dryer, use it only if you have long hair. Never use it to blow dry the short hair on your head. If you must blow dry your hair, keep the blow drier well away from your head. Not only is the heat bad for your head, but the drone of the drier can also induce a headache.

7. Avoid Pollutants

Stay away from rain - especially the first shower of the season. It is not good to let the rain fall directly on your head. Rain water may be refreshing but in can result in a headache. If you get wet in the rain, make it a point to dry your head as soon as you can. The first rains especially are very bad because the water will contain a lot of pollutants and this itself can result in a lot of diseases.

Avoid inhaling polluting gases like automobile fumes and second-hand smoking. Many of the gases let out by automobiles and other exhaust pipes are highly toxic and they itself can cause a headache. Second hand smoking by which you inhale the smoke from your neighbor's cigarette too can cause a headache. This is especially true if you are a non-smoker and not used to the smell smoke.

8. Get a Good Night's Sleep

Try to get a good night's sleep. A good night's sleep is very important to keep away headaches. "Sleep is one of the most basic and universal activities in which we all engage. Yet, getting to sleep, staying asleep, and waking refreshed can be highly elusive to most of us some of the time, and many of us all of the time." The National Sleep Foundation reports (2002) that America is on the verge of a poor sleep epidemic, characterized by the following eye-opening statistics:

- 64% of American adults get less than the eight hours of sleep that experts recommend is required to maintain optimal physical, mental, and emotional health.

- One-third of the US population says they get less sleep now than they did five years ago

- One-half of Americans have experienced insomnia (sleeplessness)

- Drowsiness due to a lack of a proper night of sleep interferes with the daily activities of 37 percent of all adults.

You need peace and quiet to get enough sleep and so you should take care to see that there are no physical disturbances. Turn the ring tone of your telephone to the lowest possible volume. Do not worry about important calls; if the calls are so important, then the caller will call back later when you have turned up the volume. Try to cut out other disturbances by wearing ear muffs or eye blinds. Do not read in bed before you sleep, in all likelihood you will drift off to sleep with the lights on and after sometime the same light will wake you up.

Do not oversleep. Oversleeping is just as bad as not getting enough sleep. If you sleep too much or for too long, you will wake up with a very woozy feeling and that will most likely turn into a headache. Our body tells us when it has had enough sleep. Listen to the cue and get up, do not succumb to the temptation to just lie in bed. Try to get at least eight hours of sleep every night. Studies have shown that this is the requirement for most healthy adults.

Examine your daily schedule to see how you can rearrange your day to ensure the right amount of sleep. Try to cut out television and other non-necessary activities.

9. Believe in Therapy

Touch therapy is a new technique that is just becoming available to cure headaches. A lot of research is going on this area and even now experts have not been able to identify how touch therapy can help in healing. The best possible explanation is that our bodies are in fact tuned to respond to the touches of others.

When we were babies our mother's touch was perhaps the most reassuring thing in the world. In fact experts are baffled by the way new born babies are able to distinguish between a mother's touch and the touch of a stranger. As we grow older we delight in the encouraging pats and caresses of our parents and teachers. Even in our social life there is a lot of touching going on. That is probably why people use the hand shake as an exchange of warmth.

So when a person is ill and miserable, the touch of another person especially if it is a person who really cares for you can relieve you of your pain. The only thing that the person has to do is to be gentle. He or she should stop when the patient has had enough.

10.   Avoid Noise

Too much noise is bad for you. In fact sound pollution is one of the causes for headaches to become so prevalent. Contrary to popular belief, sound pollution is not cause just by machines and automobiles. I do not want to argue with the fact that machines and automobiles cause a lot of sound. A journey down the street during the rush hour is enough to give anybody a headache. But apart from that blaring music too does a lot of harm.

Take care to lower the volume if you want to listen to music. Loud music is not really good for you. And if you want to play music in order to soothe your nerves and instead you are playing loud music, it will have just the opposite effect. Your blood pressure will actually go up and your adrenalin levels too will increase. The best thing that you can do is stay away from all sources of loud noise and that includes noisy kids as well.

Plug your ears if you are moving into a loud sound zone. Use ear plugs, ear muffs or thick wads of cotton. Most grocery stores and convenience stores carry sound reducing and sound-blocking earplugs, many of which are not too noticeable.

11.   Quit Smoking

Quit smoking if you can. Smoking can affect your head in a very bad way. In fact smoking affects the functioning of every part of your body. When you smoke you are actually submitting your body and the various mechanisms that go on to the power of a very strong alkaloid that is nicotine. So if you can quit smoking by all means do. It will help you live a better life and can contribute much towards eliminating your headache. In fact, if your headache goes away when you start smoking it means that your body has already become dependent on nicotine. In that case your headache may be a withdrawal symptom. There are many things that are identified with substance abuse.

Alcohol is one of them, narcotic drugs are another and tobacco is in no way to be left behind. The problem, or let us say that the similarity among all these substances is that once one gets used to them, breaking away is not easy. Contrary to popular belief, it is not the fear of deprivation of the pleasantly high feeling that drives the person to use the substance again and again so that it is used, misused and eventually abused. The person returns for his or her daily shot because of certain altered conditions in the body. These substances are indeed very potent and they affect certain specific spots or centers of the brain.

The brain quickly gets used to these alterations and then before we know it, these centers of the brain cannot do without the daily dose of the substance. The brain did not ask for the substance in the first place but we gave them to it. When we experience that pleasantly high feeling we do not bother about the changes that are taking place within. It is common knowledge that the entire processes carried about in the brain are maintained by a delicate balance of the various chemical slats there. Once we start using substances like the above mentioned tobacco, narcotics and alcohol, the balance of these chemical salts gets altered.

The body as I mentioned earlier is a self-adjusting machine and so this new chemical balance is established and it takes no time for the brain cells to get adjusted to the new balance. Then when the brain cells do not get what is required to maintain the new balance (read that as the daily puffs) things go hay wire. The old balance was disturbed and altered and a new balance was set up. But this new balance is not the real natural thing. It is something that has to be artificially supported and when that daily, or timely dose of nicotine does not get to the brain, the new balance gets upset.

12.   Drink Plenty of Water

Drink plenty of water. Water is the most important substance that your body needs. If you are not drinking enough water, you may suffer from a dehydration headache. For a person to remain healthy he or she must drink at least ten glasses of water a day. If your intake of water is less than this then by all means drink more water. Water is indeed the elixir of life. The more water you drink, the better you will feel. If you do not drink enough water, the water balance of the body will be completely disrupted. Make no mistake about this. The major content of all the cells in your body is indeed water. And when your body does not get enough water, it will end up dehydrated. This will invariably result in a headache.

ABOUT THE AUTHOR

Anne Higgins is a health advocate, a retired professor, a social entrepreneur and a writer.

A New Yorker from birth, Anne and her four sisters were raised by their widowed mother. Despite living from paycheck to paycheck, Anne graduated with the highest academic honors in high school. This earned her ticket to a college scholarship at MIT.

After her bachelor degree, Anne worked at the university hospital as a nursing assistant. While working, she enrolled and studied medicine and eventually became a doctor.

Anne is committed to helping the community by empowering members of the powers of alternative medicine.

www.ingramcontent.com/pod-product-compliance
Lightning Source LLC
Chambersburg PA
CBHW050702250726
48662CB00002B/799